CAREERS IN
PUBLIC HEALTH NURSING

REGISTERED NURSE (RN)

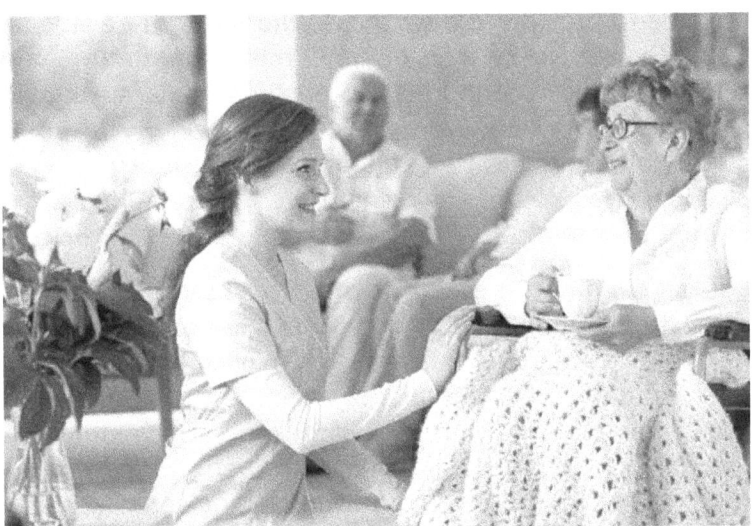

THE AMERICAN PUBLIC HEALTH ASSOCIATION defines public health nursing as the practice of promoting and protecting the health of populations using knowledge from nursing, social, and public health sciences. The core focus of the public health nursing practice focuses on promoting health and preventing disease and disability.

These specialized nurses are, in essence, responsible for ensuring the health of the whole nation. While most nurses care for one patient at a time, public health nurses (PHNs) care for entire populations. By working with whole communities, they are able to educate people about health issues, improve community health and safety, and increase access to care.

Public health nurses work on the front lines to promote and improve health. Instead of being stationed in a hospital, PHNs reach out to people in the community. This allows them to assess their environment, available resources, and potential healthcare needs. By serving individuals and families in their own environment, they are able to provide care for those who may not be able to obtain healthcare services by other means. In group settings such as community centers or workplaces, they stop the spread of disease, prevent injury, and ward off illness through education and direct intervention. They also keep people safer by helping them prepare for natural disasters.

Public health nurses comprise the largest segment of the professional public health workforce and serve in many different critical roles. Public health may conjure images of community medical clinics or awareness campaigns promoting healthy living. It is all that, but much more. The public health nurse is expected to perform many functions beyond providing quality nursing care, such as collaborating with community agencies and elected officials, monitoring emerging epidemics, helping to develop better healthcare policy, and participating in legislative movements.

PHNs work in a variety of settings such as health departments, schools, homes, community health centers, clinics, correctional facilities, work sites, and out of mobile vans. Where they work often determines their roles and responsibilities. For example, a PHN working in a community health clinic might provide immunizations and medical treatments, manage wellness clinics, and help people dealing with violence, pregnancy, or substance abuse. Within a government agency, the work would involve researching potential health epidemics and how to mitigate them. In a remote village in an undeveloped country, a PHN would work to slow a pandemic or reduce infant mortality through education.

Public health nursing is generally considered a specialized field of registered nursing, which usually means a four-year Bachelor of Science in Nursing (BSN) degree is required. Because there is a nursing shortage that shows no signs of letting up, it is possible to start with a two-year Associate Degree in Nursing (ADN) that is available at most community colleges. About half of all public health nurses enter the profession with an ADN, but nearly all eventually obtain a BSN because it is needed to qualify for jobs with more responsibility, advancement opportunities, and higher salaries. Many employers help their nurses obtain a BSN, offering tuition assistance and flexible scheduling so these nurses can continue to work while going back to school.

Entry-level public health nurses start out earning on average $50,000 a year. After a few years of experience and earning a BSN, the average rises to $70,000. There are other nursing fields that offer higher pay, but none provides greater overall job satisfaction. In addition to the opportunity to improve the lives of great numbers of people, PHNs enjoy great benefits packages, exceptional autonomy, normal working hours, and good work/life balance. Plus, they can count on job security since robust job growth is expected, with more public health nurses needed each year for the foreseeable future. Nurses have many options, but if you want a broader, fuller life, public health nursing can be a great choice.

WHAT YOU CAN DO NOW

IN HIGH SCHOOL, MAKE SURE YOU TAKE the classes that you will need to be admitted to a college with a nursing program. This typically means four years of higher level math, science, and English classes. Take as many Advanced Placement (AP) classes as possible, especially in math and science subjects. The more you learn in high school, the better your chances of success in college. Learn and practice good study, organizational, and test taking skills and maintain a high GPA. Nursing program admissions are based largely on GPA and college entrance exam scores.

If you are good at taking tests or are especially advanced in some subjects, consider taking the College Level Examination Program (CLEP) tests. Passing a CLEP test means you can skip that class in college, which saves time and money. There are 33 different subjects that are eligible for college credits, but each college has its own policy regarding which ones are accepted. Ask your high school counselor to help you determine which CLEP tests you should take.

CPR and first aid classes are required for a nursing license, but you can take them while still in high school. These classes are offered by community centers, fire departments, and the American Red Cross. Getting your certifications out of the way now will give you a head start in nursing school.

Get some real experience in nursing through volunteer work. It is a great way to test out this career before making a long-term commitment. It will add weight to your nursing school application and get your résumé off to a good start. Community health centers and other medical facilities always need a helping hand. The need is so great, in fact, that you can find tons of opportunities with a simple Web search. Some hospitals even offer summer volunteer programs specifically for high school students. You can also get practice by working with a local neighborhood association, home health provider, or hospice. If you think you might be interested in focusing on public health policy, offer a helping hand to a health advocacy group.

Join HOSA-Future Health Professionals if it is available at your school. It is an instructional program designed to prepare students for a future in the healthcare industry.

HISTORY OF THE CAREER

PREVENTIVE CARE AND CURATIVE CARE have gone hand in hand since ancient times. In Greek mythology, Hygeia was the goddess of preventive health while her sister Panacea was the goddess of healing. However, prevention took a back seat to treating those already sick for many centuries. It was not until the mid-19th century that this attitude began to change in a meaningful way.

By 1850, the medical community had become more interested in finding the causes of disease. Autopsies became more common and many doctors started collecting data that might provide clues. One such doctor was Hungarian physician, Ignaz Semmelweis. While working in a maternity ward in Vienna, he noticed a difference in the mortality rate between the ward staffed by doctors and the ward staffed by midwives. His data showed that women in the ward staffed by doctors died at a rate nearly five times higher than those in the midwives' clinic. It was widely believed that the women died of "childbed fever," a malady of unknown origin. He considered a number of theories, all of which proved false.

At the time, doctors routinely performed autopsies on women who died in the hospital. When one of these doctors died, Semmelweis realized that he had died of the same thing as the women he had autopsied. He hypothesized that particles from cadavers were getting on the hands of the pathologists and were transferred to the insides of women during delivery. His correct conclusion was that getting rid of the cadaverous particles would cut down the death rate. The medical staff was ordered to start cleaning their hands and instruments with the best disinfectant known, which was chlorine. The rate of death fell dramatically. Without knowing anything about germs, Semmelweis had discovered that hand-washing is one of the most important tools in public health. It can keep kids from getting the flu from classmates, and hospitalized patients from contracting life-threatening infections.

This new understanding of how sanitation interventions could prevent disease on a large scale was initially shunned by physicians. However, preventive care was carried forward in England as district nursing became the first role for public health nurses. At the same time, Florence Nightingale was making it her mission to improve hygiene practices in order to lower the death rate in hospitals. Her greatest success came during the Crimean War, where 18,000 soldiers were admitted to military hospitals. In 1854, Nightingale organized a team of 34 nurses to tend to the sick and fallen soldiers. What they found when they arrived at the British base hospital in Constantinople was appalling. The hospital sat on top of a large cesspool, which contaminated the water and the hospital building itself. Rodents and bugs were everywhere. Basics, like bandages and soap, were scarce. More soldiers were dying from infectious diseases than from injuries suffered in battle.

Nightingale ordered the hospital to be scrubbed top to bottom. Bedding was sanitized and clean water was brought in. Food meeting special dietary and nutrition requirements was cooked. The result was a reduction in the hospital's death rate by two-thirds. Based on this experience, Nightingale wrote an 830-page report, *Notes on Matters Affecting the Health, Efficiency and Hospital Administration of the British Army*, that proposed reforms for other military hospitals operating under poor conditions. The book also led to the establishment of a Royal Commission for the Health of the Army in 1857.

The term "public health nurse" was coined by Lillian Wald. She was the first to propose that public health nursing should involve the health of an entire neighborhood. Wald and Mary Brewster, both graduates of the New York Hospital School of Nursing, moved to the Lower East Side of New York City to put this concept of public health nursing into practice. It was 1893 and the 19th century's worst depression was underway. They went throughout the neighborhood, giving patients ice, sterilized milk, meals, medicines, and referrals to hospitals and dispensaries. Wald and Brewster soon moved out of their tenement building and into a house that became known as the Henry Street Nurses' Settlement. The house was soon inhabited by nurses, activists, lawyers, union organizers, and social reformers.

A number of prominent philanthropists supported the Henry Street Settlement activities, and the enterprise grew dramatically with additional houses opening throughout the city. By the early 1900s, Wald's vision had led to public health nursing roles being extended beyond the care of the sick to encompass advocacy, community organizing, health education, and political reform. Public health nursing in the United States and other countries quickly grew to include working in diverse settings, such as public and private hospitals, communities, prisons, homes, schools, neighborhoods, and work sites. By 1910, most of the large visiting nurses associations and numerous boards of health and education had initiated disease-prevention programs.

By the late 1920s, public health nursing had evolved into a separate, specialized field. Thousands of small and independent local government and voluntary agencies were sponsoring public health nurses. This was proving to be inefficient, as there were many gaps and duplications in services. Many nursing leaders advocated for the creation of comprehensive, coordinated public nursing services. Numerous studies and demonstration projects from the 1920s through the 1940s confirmed that such a system would better meet the needs of most of the public who needed these services. Public health nursing, as a distinct nursing specialty, gave rise to population-oriented, preventive health care for all.

Over the years, public health nurses have assumed a variety of roles and titles, but many challenges lie ahead. Today, they are faced with frightening diseases that can affect millions. There are numerous environmental hazards. The alienation among the disenfranchised has continued to create unmet health needs of populations at greatest risk. Some believe there is a crisis in caring. Many believe there needs to be a major paradigm shift in public health policy. Both may be right. The need is great for public health nurses to help turn an inadequate medical care system into a healthcare system that provides for all the public.

WHERE YOU WILL WORK

PUBLIC HEALTH NURSES WORK MORE WITH entire communities than with individuals. Because their focus is on disease prevention and advocating for better health through education and lifestyle changes, they are not like typical nurses waiting for patients to come to the hospital when they are sick. Instead they go out into communities to do their work. Many do choose to stay in hospital settings or clinics. However, they are most often found in public health agencies, which may be privately owned or run by the city, county, or state department of health. There are also positions in federal government agencies that deal with health-related issues.

There are many other work settings besides public health departments. Where any individual PHN will work depends on that person's training, experience, and interests. It could be anything from an occupational health facility to a correctional facility.

PHNs who want to work directly with members of the community on a range of health concerns are often situated in community clinics. In this environment, they can usually order tests and sometimes even prescribe medication without a doctor's direct supervision. Some work in outpatient clinics, which are different in that they are typically associated with a hospital. Outpatient clinics are often focused on a particular type of patient or health concern, such as elderly people, opioid addiction, or AIDS.

Education is at the heart of public health nursing work. PHNs often give presentations at senior centers, community groups, schools, or wherever they need to inform people about important health and safety issues. It is particularly necessary to reach children early so they understand how to maintain their own health and prevent illnesses. PHNs often work in schools, where they deal with a variety of issues and teach children about nutrition, exercise, hygiene, sexual health, and preventing the spread of various illnesses.

There are also numerous nonprofit organizations that hire large numbers of public health nurses. Most of these organizations focus on delivering health information and solutions for people in significantly disenfranchised communities. Some of the best-known include the Red Cross, the Peace Corps, and Doctors Without Borders, but these are just a few among many.

PHNs are most needed in rural and low-income communities, anywhere that lack sufficient healthcare providers. In underserved areas, they provide critical services, such as immunizing school children, providing prenatal and well-baby care, and teaching the elderly how to stay safe and healthy at home.

Public health nurses practice in diverse settings, such as housing developments, neighborhood centers, parishes, and worksites. They tend to move around rather than stay situated in a central location. In many cases, they provide services from mobile units that may be called in to respond to potential health crises. They also may travel locally or to other regions to have meetings with stakeholders, government officials, or community groups. Some go directly to people's homes. Public health nurses can also work privately or on a consulting basis.

THE WORK YOU WILL DO

PUBLIC HEALTH NURSING IS A VERY UNIQUE specialization in the registered nursing field. Public health nurses provide education and a wide array of services that support healthy people and communities. The most common tasks include educating the public about preventive medicine, running wellness clinics, treating patients in public health clinics, and working with youth in schools and community centers.

Many public health nurses work in government offices. Those working in city and county health departments run clinics, provide healthcare and nutritional services for pregnant women and children, administer screening tests to identify infectious diseases, provide immunizations, and work to provide better access to healthcare for low-income and other underserved people such as immigrants and those living in remote areas. At the federal level, PHNs identify and track patterns of illness and other health trends in order to develop programs that address and contain disease outbreaks and generally promote health nationwide.

Some public health nurses work in hospitals where they develop and teach classes on various topics, such as newborn care, CPR, smoking cessation, and nutrition, that promotes better health. There are many PHNs working in areas where there are no hospitals. They often use mobile units to reach people who need healthcare services in places where there are no conventional medical facilities.

Most nurses care for individual patients that come to them after being injured or getting sick. Public health nursing is different. PHNs are responsible for the health of an entire population. By working with whole communities, they can help stop diseases from spreading, boost overall community safety and health, develop emergency plans to respond to natural disasters, and provide medical information that people might otherwise never know.

Public health nurses work with many different types of populations besides neighborhoods and communities. For example, they may be employed in schools, teaching children about preventing head lice or helping teens deal with stress and improve their sexual and reproductive health. They might help pregnant women and new mothers get access to more nutritious foods or deal with breast feeding issues. They might work in prisons, helping to maintain the health and safety of inmates. They also might be responsible for workplace safety, inspecting workplaces for safety risks and formulating plans for increasing worker safety and improving health.

Public Health Nursing Roles

Public health nursing can be difficult to define because it encompasses so many different roles. At the most basic level, it might involve providing medical care in an impoverished urban neighborhood. At an overall level, it can have global repercussions by preventing epidemics and improving the health of entire nations. In between is an incredibly diverse array of roles that fall under the umbrella of public health nursing. These may include the familiar jobs of monitoring health hazards unique to certain communities, to more indirect career options such as working with marketing professionals to develop wellness campaigns or helping law enforcement officials focus on substance abuse prevention rather than punishment.

What any public health nurse does depends on a variety of factors. It is typical to specialize in a particular kind of practice, which may refer to the type of work, where the work is done, or who the employer is. The most common focus of public health nurses is health education. In fact, public health nurses focus more on education and prevention than any single task.

Some public health nurses work to improve the overall health and well-being of an entire group or population through education. They do this through presentations at schools, community groups, senior centers, and other local groups. The central theme might be proper nutrition, effective safety practices, early detection of common diseases, or other important health issues.

Other public health nurses provide educational services for high-risk individuals. For example, when working with addicts and sex workers, they would encourage certain behaviors that would prevent overdoses or the spread of disease. For the general population, they might provide nutritional information to individuals and help them access and choose healthy, economical foods. A better diet is a powerful tool in decreasing rates of malnutrition, obesity, and illnesses that stem from poor nutrition.

Many public health nurses spend their entire careers working in low-income or rural areas, both here and in undeveloped countries. Their services are critical to the health and well-being of people in these areas. Many patients in underserved, rural, or underprivileged communities do not get any healthcare at all, either because there are no medical providers or they cannot afford the available care.

The working conditions in these areas are often difficult and the needs are great. PHNs are sometimes the only healthcare professionals for miles around to educate and treat patients and families in need. They typically have minimal budgets and sometimes there is not even a dedicated space to work in, yet there is a long list of responsibilities and tasks to attend to. At the very least, they need to immunize school children, provide prenatal and well-baby care, and teach the elderly how to stay safe and healthy at home. They also need to constantly monitor the community for signs of potential health crises and respond to infectious disease outbreaks. They often act as a role model to the community, which is often the best way to teach and motivate members of the community to adopt healthy behaviors and lifestyles.

Advanced Public Health Nursing Roles

Some public health nurses who work for the government specialize in disaster preparedness and response. This is a type of practice that requires additional training and certification. In this role, public health nurses facilitate catastrophic event planning, and manage and provide resources in response to a wide array of threats to community safety. An emergency response may be triggered by natural disasters, communicable disease outbreaks, or civil problems, such as water pollution.

At the federal level, PHNs in this role are often an important part of the National Preparedness System, which is run by FEMA. They participate in four different disaster stages, including prevention, preparedness, response, and recovery. The PHNs are trained in all four stages, but may be assigned to one. For example, in the first stage they might work on developing plans to educate the public about what to do during an evacuation to prevent unnecessary injuries. A nurse in the response stage, however, would work on triaging victims and determining what resources the community needs.

Government employed public health nurses may also be involved in research. This often requires graduate school training. Research is important because the data that researchers collect are used to validate funding for public health programs, reduce inequalities in healthcare, and increase access to services. PHNs in this role may monitor health trends in certain communities in order to determine how to improve community health or evaluate how some initiatives have performed. For example, public health nurses may determine whether mobile clinics have improved the outcomes for mothers giving birth in underserved communities.

STORIES OF PUBLIC HEALTH NURSES

I Work in an Inner City Health Clinic

"This clinic is a designated primary care setting located in a disadvantaged neighborhood. Our goal is to meet the needs of a full spectrum of the population from birth to old age. The work we do covers a lot of ground from wound care to palliative care, so teamwork is essential. We each have specific roles, but we often need to help each other. My focus is on prenatal and early childhood.

A day in the life of any PHN is never dull and always brings new challenges. The day starts with a team meeting before making home visits to newborn infants to do neonatal screening and follow up on hospital referrals. Back in the clinic I lead the breast feeding support group, manage the drop-in clinic for expectant parents, perform early child health and development screenings, and run parenting courses.

The best part of my job is getting to know the families. It puts me in a better position to treat my patients holistically. I also like the autonomy. Unlike most nurses, I decide what my clients need, and I can be innovative in meeting those needs. I'm not crazy about the paperwork. There is a lot of it, and when the weather is bad, I still have to go out and make my home visits. But those are minor complaints.

Nurses can choose from an extraordinary array of specializations. I didn't know I wanted to be a PHN until I interned for a home health agency. I found that nursing people in their own environment was more comfortable than a hospital setting for both me and my patients. You may see it differently, but you won't know unless you try it."

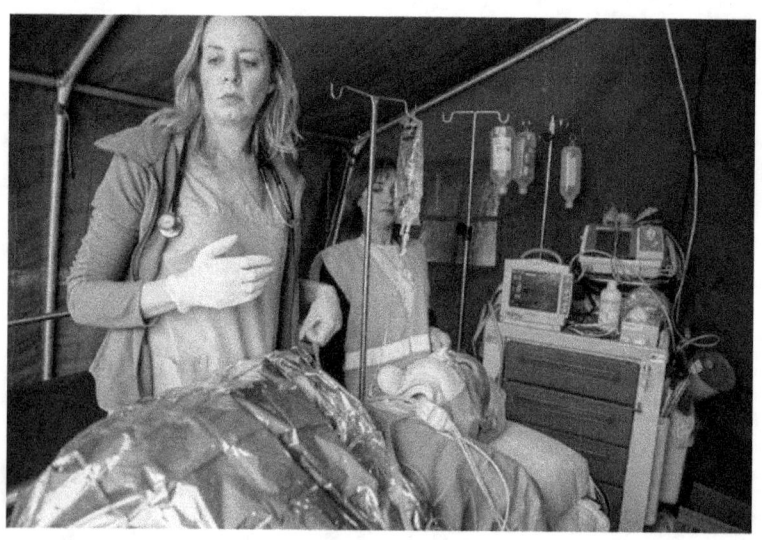

I Am Certified in Disaster Management

"Most people think disaster nursing is all about adrenaline pumping drama. That can be the case during major events like massive wildfires and hurricanes. There may be thousands of displaced patients, some needing dialysis, others suffering from critical wounds, and everyone is scared. It can be an overwhelming experience. But after the initial response, the primary goal in a widespread disaster is to keep the daily routine going. In addition to emergency services, medical facilities still need to be provided, homebound patients still need caregivers, and babies are still being born. The usual nursing staff is often unable to get to work, which means double and triple shifts for those who can. Despite the best planning, you may run out of supplies and the electricity may fail. I help nurses think creatively about how they could make do with diminishing resources. All in all, it's tough, exhausting work, and absolutely the best job in the world!

A disaster PHN has many roles to fill, and much of the work is done before an event occurs. Disasters happen infrequently. I live in a Gulf state where the hurricane season lasts six months a year. I spend most of my off-season time developing response plans for facilities, training regular nursing staff in how to follow their institution's disaster plan, consulting with home health agencies, and advising employers on how to protect their workers.

I am also responsible for community preparedness. It is natural to think bad things only happen to someone else, and my job is to convince people to prepare for the worst case scenario. I show them what goes into a jump kit – solar-powered flashlight, portable rechargers for phones, wind-up radio, insurance policy numbers, medications, water, and food. I also help families determine their own escape routes and designated place to reunite. It seems simple, but it saves lives.

The nation is experiencing more storms and fires than ever, and they are bigger and more dangerous than ever. We need more PHNs to help with mitigation, preparation, response, and recovery.

My advice for anyone considering public health nursing is to start by volunteering. Visit the website of NVOAD (National Association of Voluntary Organizations) to find where you are needed most. Even if you don't decide to continue in this area, with the necessary training and certification, the experience will change your life. I know it has made me a better person and nurse."

PERSONAL QUALIFICATIONS

PUBLIC HEALTH NURSES ARE HIGHLY dedicated professionals who are passionate about improving community health and safety through education, public policy, and large scale preventive measures. Every PHN prepares for this career by getting proper training. There are also some personal characteristics that the most successful PHNs share in common. These traits are not learned in a classroom, but can be developed and nurtured as you gain experience in the field.

Because public health nursing is focused on disseminating information, strong communications skills are essential. All day, every day, PHNs are discussing healthcare practices directly with individual patients, groups, or entire populations. They also work with a variety of other professionals, including caregivers, physicians, community organizers, and government public health policymakers. Excellent speaking skills are needed to convey important information in a way that a particular individual or group can easily understand and act on. It is also important to be a good listener and effective teacher.

Because public health nurses are concerned with many different people, excellent interpersonal skills are needed. PHNs need to be able to quickly establish rapport and trust so people will accept what they are being told. You will need to be patient, understanding, and observant in order to know what kind of information is needed. It is especially important to be broad-minded and nonjudgmental. You must be sensitive to cultural differences and lifestyle issues that might be affecting a person's health and safety.

Good organizational skills are also important for keeping track of information and maintaining proper records. Public health nurses usually have a variety of responsibilities and may be working on multiple tasks or issues at the same time. It takes discipline and good time management to stay on top of it all.

Money management skills are helpful, too. PHNs often have to deal with scarce resources and budget restrictions. The most successful PHNs are able to manage resources effectively by focusing efforts where they will do the most good.

In many instances, public health nurses are working on their own to develop solutions to problems. Critical thinking is needed, especially when working in the homes of patients or in isolated areas far from the resources of a well-equipped medical facility. The best PHNs are able to make decisions on the spot about a person's or community's health status or needs. They are independent thinkers who are able to work on their own without the constant supervision most nurses experience.

ATTRACTIVE FEATURES

MOST PEOPLE GO INTO NURSING because they genuinely want to help people. Few nursing fields provide the opportunities to help others as much as public health nursing does. PHNs report great satisfaction with their careers because they can impact the health and safety of so many people at once, rather than care for one person at a time who is already sick. Plus, there are many settings to choose from. Whether in a community clinic, small rural town, school, government agency, or a faraway country, PHNs have extraordinary opportunities to contribute to people's lives and well-being, and to create social change.

The level of autonomy in public health nursing is much higher than that of other nursing fields. Most nurses work under supervision and can only do what doctors or charge nurses direct them to do. PHNs work independently most of the time. This allows plenty of room for your own fresh ideas and initiatives. You can design new materials and procedures, create your own outreach program, determine how your resources will be used, and make your own schedule.

A career in public health nursing is relatively easy to get into. Although most PHNs earn a bachelor's degree, it is possible to obtain the training necessary to qualify for an entry-level public nursing position in as few as 18 months. Many employers help their nurses earn their bachelor's degree while still working, with tuition and scheduling assistance. Regardless of the training they start with, nurses in public health are assured of having secure jobs.

Nurses in general are exceptionally hard workers. They are often scheduled to work 12 hour shifts, plus overtime and holidays. Public health nursing is very different. They usually work regular hours with no overtime, weekends, or holidays required. Plus, they can often manage their own schedules.

Public health nurses usually enjoy very generous benefit packages. While there are higher paying salaries in other nursing fields, the benefits can partially compensate for the difference. This is because so many PHNs are employed by federal, state, and local government agencies. In some cases, they are eligible for lucrative retirement programs after as few as 10 years.

For many PHNs, the work is all about the people they help. Most of us will probably never get to know people in rural communities or impoverished urban neighborhoods. Public health nurses get to meet and work with all kinds of people with very diverse backgrounds and unique stories. Meeting them provides a better understanding of humanity in general and health issues in particular.

UNATTRACTIVE ASPECTS

A CAREER IN PUBLIC HEALTH NURSING is not for everyone. While it has much to offer, it does have some negatives. The pay is better in other nursing fields. The paperwork can be daunting. The working environments can be unpleasant or downright primitive. There are other downsides that should be considered before planning for a future public health nursing career.

Public health nurses are dedicated to improving community health and access to care. It takes hard work and a long time to accomplish that. Underserved communities, whether in rural areas or in poor urban neighborhoods, usually have a long history of health problems within their populations. Community members may be suffering from multiple acute and chronic conditions. It is not easy to remove systemic barriers to healthcare, deal with environmental pollutants, improve nutrition, and teach people healthy behaviors. Some factors, such as remoteness or culture, cannot be overcome. PHNs have to know their own limits so they do not burn out. In order to succeed, you will need to be patient and understand that it can take years to make meaningful progress.

One of the main reasons for poor health in communities is lack of resources. Public health departments and nonprofit organizations do what they can, but they usually have limited funds. You may not have the space or facilities to offer clinical services, or enough supplies to provide treatments. There may be no money to hire paid staff or even to create educational materials. The most successful PHNs are resourceful. They allocate their scarce resources wisely and find creative ways to get what is needed most.

Public health is often one of the first services to be cut when budgets are squeezed. To avoid being laid off, look for stable positions that are well funded and less likely to come to a sudden end. For example, a position with a larger healthcare provider is more likely to last than one with a state agency. If you are not sure about the longevity of a position, it is okay to ask what the outlook is during an interview. The alternative is to make sure you get some hospital experience before going into the public health field so you have something to fall back on if your job gets cut.

EDUCATION AND TRAINING

PUBLIC HEALTH NURSING IS GENERALLY considered a specialized field of Registered Nursing, for which a four-year Bachelor of Science in Nursing (BSN) degree is usually required. However, due to the increasing need for qualified nurses, an Associate Degree in Nursing (ADN) is enough to qualify for many entry-level public health jobs in hospitals, outpatient clinics, and home health agencies. ADN programs typically last only two years, include clinical experience, and are available at most community colleges. In most states, you can work as an RN with an associate degree. In fact, nearly half of RN licenses are obtained initially through ADN programs.

Nurses with a BSN are eligible for jobs with more responsibility, advancement opportunities, and higher salaries. Many employers help their nurses obtain BSNs offering tuition assistance and flexible scheduling so these nurses can continue to work while going back to school.

ADN and BSN programs follow the same core curriculum that includes courses like anatomy, biology, chemistry, as well as practical nursing courses in adult health, maternal and newborn nursing, and pediatrics. Some programs also include psychiatric nursing, community health nursing, and gerontological nursing.

A BSN program builds on the core curriculum with more advanced courses like microbiology, physiology, and organic chemistry.

Courses specific to the practice of nursing may include subjects like nursing theory and nursing research. A popular new addition to most programs is nursing informatics, which is a field of study that examines how nurses use technology.

Students who already have a degree in a field other than nursing can transfer to a BSN degree, often at an accelerated rate. Accelerated programs can take anywhere from 18 months (if going full time with no breaks between semesters) to two years. Clinical requirements are the same as those of full four-year BSN programs. Admission standards are higher though, with a 3.0 GPA minimum required for admission. Some programs also have prerequisites such as human anatomy and physiology, chemistry with a lab component, nutrition, statistics, microbiology, and developmental psychology.

While in college, students should look for opportunities to learn more about public health issues. Consider seeking additional training in public health, public policy, health administration, and related subjects. Find ways to work in community health environments, health advocacy groups, or wherever you can get experience in the field.

Once you have completed your training, you will need to get licensed before you can practice as a nurse. Public health nurses must take and pass the national NCLEX-RN examination, available from state nursing boards. This qualifies them as a Registered Nurse. Some states also require passage of a Public Health or Community Health Nursing Certification Exam. Before taking those exams, you need to work for at least 500 hours in a public health position as an RN in order to obtain the needed experience. Additional training might be necessary in specific facilities and states as well.

Certain public health nursing jobs, such as leadership roles and research, require graduate education. Master of Science in Nursing (MSN), Doctor of Nursing Practice (DNP), and Doctor of Philosophy (PhD) degrees qualify nurses for advanced positions in public health nursing.

There is also an Advanced Public Health Nurse-Board Certified (APHN-BC) credential offered by the American Nurses Credentialing Center. Unlike the state-issued licenses, this certification does not require an examination. Instead, it is awarded via portfolio submission. Eligibility criteria include:

- Minimum of two years practice as an RN full time
- Minimum of 2,000 hours practicing in the specialty of advanced public health nursing within the past three years
- Hold a BSN plus a graduate degree in nursing or a graduate degree in public health
- Minimum of 30 continuing education units in advanced public health related to nursing within the past three years
- Additional evidence of exceptional professional development

EARNINGS

THERE ARE BETTER PAYING NURSING JOBS, but most public health nurses go into this field for the intangible rewards. According to the American Public Health Association, the average yearly salary for public health nurses is about $70,000. There are also usually bonuses averaging $2,500. Some PHNs also get overtime pay, but that is less common in this specialization. The range is fairly wide with the lowest 10 percent of salaries in the $50,000 range, and the highest 10 percent earning more than $85,000. Salaries vary by experience, job location, and type of position.

Starting out, an entry-level PHN with fewer than five years of experience can expect to earn an average total compensation of $50,000. That includes salary, bonuses, and overtime pay. Most PHNs who remain in the field until they are mid-career, will reach the overall national average of $70,000. Earning more will require additional education, specialized training, or experience in management.

The biggest differences in salaries are associated with location. In fact, a public health nurse can earn twice as much in Washington, DC as in Hawaii. Washington, DC leads the nation with PHNs earning an average of $80,000. Other states paying well above the national average include New York, Georgia, Connecticut, New Jersey, and Missouri. Salaries in these states are in the $75,000 range. At the other end of the scale are states paying less than the national average, such as Idaho and Alaska. In these states PHN salaries average $45,000.

In many fields, jobs in rural areas pay less than those in dense population areas, but in public health nursing, that is not necessarily the case. Rural states like Mississippi, Arkansas, and Alabama actually pay public health nurses more than the national average, while a state like Arizona pays far less, and California is in the middle.

There are many different ways you can practice public health nursing. How much you earn may depend on which one you choose. For example, you could become a research associate for a state government agency. It would probably be fascinating work, contributing to the growing body of clinical knowledge in the field of public health, but the money would not be great, with a salary of less than $40,000. Compare that to working as a health policy nurse, taking on the tasks of advocacy, research, analysis, and policy development. Not only do these nurses have the satisfaction of helping to bring better healthcare to large groups of people, or even the entire nation, they can earn anywhere from $80,000 to $140,000 a year. It requires earning a master's degree and completing a health policy residency program in a government office, advocacy organization, or community group, but if working on health policy is appealing, that additional time spent in school could be well worth it.

Most public health nurses work full time which means they usually receive good benefits. At the very least, they can expect to receive health insurance that covers medical, dental, vision, and prescriptions. Those working for the government typically receive more benefits than those in the private sector. Government employees enjoy an excellent benefits package that includes comprehensive health- care benefits, excellent retirement plans, paid holidays and vacation time, plus assorted extras like help with child and dependent care.

OPPORTUNITIES

THE FUTURE LOOKS BRIGHT FOR PUBLIC HEALTH NURSES with increasing pay rates and a growing number of job opportunities expected. Government experts estimate that job growth in this field will climb almost 20 percent over the coming decade, which is much faster than average for all other occupations. Job demand for all nurses in general is going up fast, but the need for those in the public health sector is particularly great. According to the Association of Schools of Public Health, there is a shortage of public health workers because of the constantly growing need for services in disadvantaged populations and the emergence of new biological and environmental threats to overall public health. Opportunities will continue to be heavily concentrated in rural and low-income areas here and abroad.

There are a number of other reasons for the job growth. One is the aging population, since older people generally have more medical problems than younger people. There is also the continuing rise in obesity and diabetes that require nurses to educate and care for patients with those and other chronic conditions.

Nurses in the public health field also help relieve one of the biggest problems in healthcare today – rising costs. Many government organizations have accepted that providing better preventive services not only keeps people healthier, it helps reduce overall healthcare costs. At the heart of the PHN's job is the emphasis on preventive care and promoting better public health. If, through education, diseases can be prevented from occurring in the first place, the high costs of treatment and hospitalization can be avoided. This realization has prompted more government agencies at all levels from city to federal to hire more PHNs than any other group of employers.

The profession encourages diversity in its ranks because public health nurses often work with diverse populations. Bilingual nurses, particularly those fluent in both Spanish and English, are especially needed.

Unlike other kinds of nurses, PHNs have a range of great opportunities outside of hands-on caregiving. Some of the best include the following:

- **Public health educators** are employed by numerous domestic and international organizations to fight major diseases through education. For example, a public health educator specializing in HIV/AIDS prevention might work for a nonprofit organization in a developing country, training HIV counselors and teaching educators how to help people in their communities avoid the disease.

- **Public health information officers** work for public health agencies in the US and other countries. They are responsible for disseminating accurate and timely information about public health issues. This may include getting vital information to affected areas quickly in order to reduce a community's risk in a public health emergency.

- **Project specialists in public health** fill many of the new jobs becoming available. Their work is primarily focused on developing health policies and making policy decisions that affect large populations around the world.

- **Disaster specialists** are concerned with preventing various man-made or natural disasters from growing into major public health emergencies. They develop effective disaster response initiatives and train other public health professionals and first responders in what to do in different scenarios.

- **Research associates** are needed to contribute to the growing body of clinical knowledge in the field of public health. State and local governments, international health agencies, as well as public and private foundations hire these specialists to work on basic and applied research projects. They also conduct pilot tests to determine the feasibility, acceptability, and preliminary effectiveness of proposed public health projects.

GETTING STARTED

THE NEED FOR PUBLIC HEALTH NURSES has never been greater. Once you complete your training and get your nursing license, the hardest part is over. Getting started is not at all complicated. Following some simple steps will lead you to a good job for someone starting out.

A successful job search starts with knowing what you are looking for. There are more possible work settings than you might imagine. Begin by narrowing down the possibilities – government agency or private health organization, city or country, dynamic or static environment, etc. Next, consider what kind of work is most appealing. For example, you could choose to work with a certain age group or particular health issue. You might enjoy talking to large groups or prefer working one-on-one in a person's home. You could work behind the scenes to improve supply chain management of medicines or on the front lines, diagnosing infectious diseases in poor countries.

Now that you have a clear idea of what you want, you can write a résumé that reflects your goals. Start fleshing out your résumé with as much hands-on experience as you can from internships and volunteering. There are many internships available to nurses and most of them offer good pay. It often takes time to get admitted to internship programs. Get experience by volunteering in any medical environment even if it is only for a short time. Even though you will not get paid, it looks good on a résumé because it demonstrates your professional commitment.

Network, network, network. While you are getting your experience through internships and volunteer positions, you should be building a network of contacts. Although there are many publicly advertised jobs for nurses, the best jobs usually come through personal contacts. In addition to professors and supervisors, contacts can be any professionals who are a little more senior than you. You can also make contacts at conferences sponsored by professional nursing associations. Always be reaching out to your network, letting your contacts know you are available and what you are looking for.

Take advantage of the services offered by your college career center. There you will find job postings, notices of job fairs, and scheduled visits by recruiters. Be sure to visit the career center often so you are the first in line to get an interview. You can also get help with polishing your résumé and honing your interviewing skills.

Public health nursing jobs can be found all over the internet. You can find thousands of them posted on the general job sites, but there are also many sites devoted to the healthcare industry. Some even focus solely on nursing jobs:

- NurseRecruiter.com
- IHireNursing.com
- NursingJobs.com

These industry-specific sites make it especially easy to sort through the many job posts. You can search by license type, city or state, and area of interest. Professional nursing associations also post jobs on their websites.

ASSOCIATIONS

■ **Association of Public Health Nurses**
http://www.phnurse.org

- **American Public Health Association**
  https://apha.org

- **American Nurses Credentialing Center (ANCC)**
  https://www.nursingworld.org/ancc

- **National Board of Public Health Examiners**
  https://www.nbphe.org

PERIODICALS

- **Nurse Journal**
  https://nursejournal.org

- **American Journal of Public Health**
  https://ajph.aphapublications.org/loi/ajph

WEBSITES

- www.NurseRecruiter.com

- www.IhireNursing.com

- www.NursingJobs.com

- www.PracticalNursing.org
  National Voluntary Organizations Active in Disaster (NVOAD)
  https://www.nvoad.org

Copyright 2019
Institute For Career Research
CAREERS INTERNET DATABASE
www.careers-internet.org

www.ingramcontent.com/pod-product-compliance
Lightning Source LLC
Chambersburg PA
CBHW051206170526
45158CB00005B/1844